Baby Shower For

_____

_____

Date

_____

_____

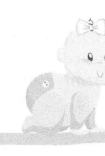

Guest Name

_____

Relationship to Parents

_____

Advice for Parents

_____

_____

_____

_____

Wishes for Baby

_____

_____

_____

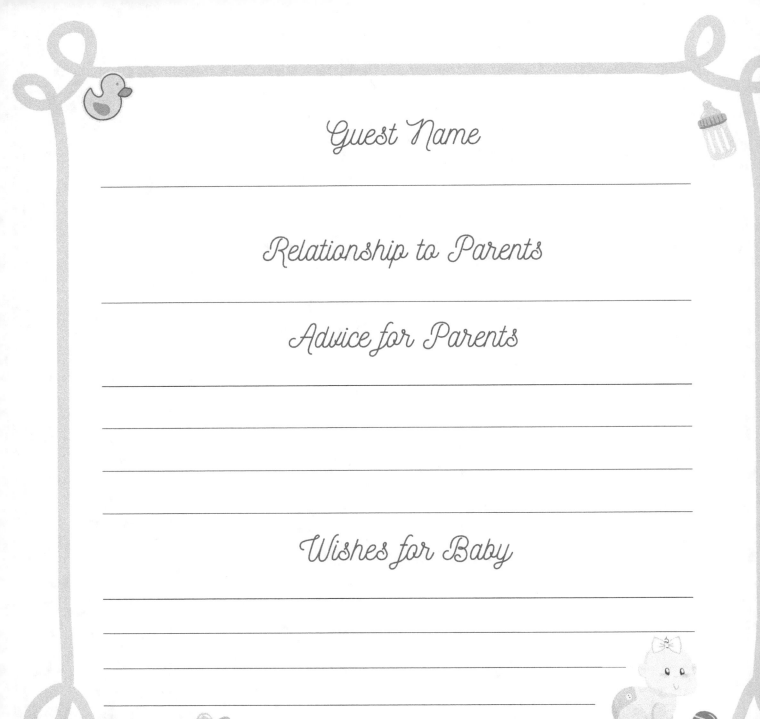

Guest Name

_____

Relationship to Parents

_____

Advice for Parents

_____

_____

_____

Wishes for Baby

_____

_____

_____

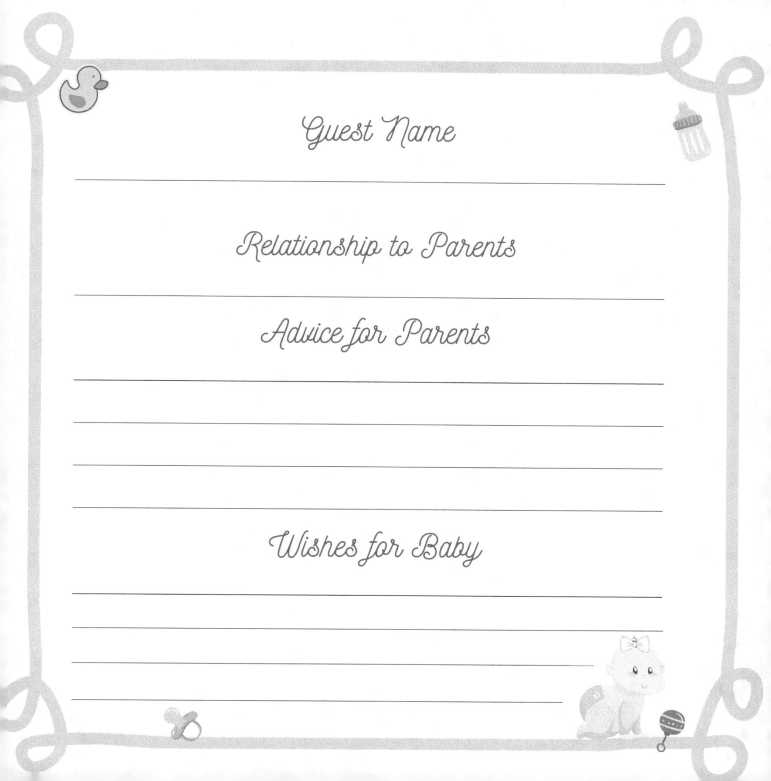

Guest Name

_____

Relationship to Parents

_____

Advice for Parents

_____

_____

_____

Wishes for Baby

_____

_____

_____

Guest Name

_____

Relationship to Parents

_____

Advice for Parents

_____

_____

_____

Wishes for Baby

_____

_____

_____

Guest Name

_____

Relationship to Parents

_____

Advice for Parents

_____

_____

_____

Wishes for Baby

_____

_____

_____

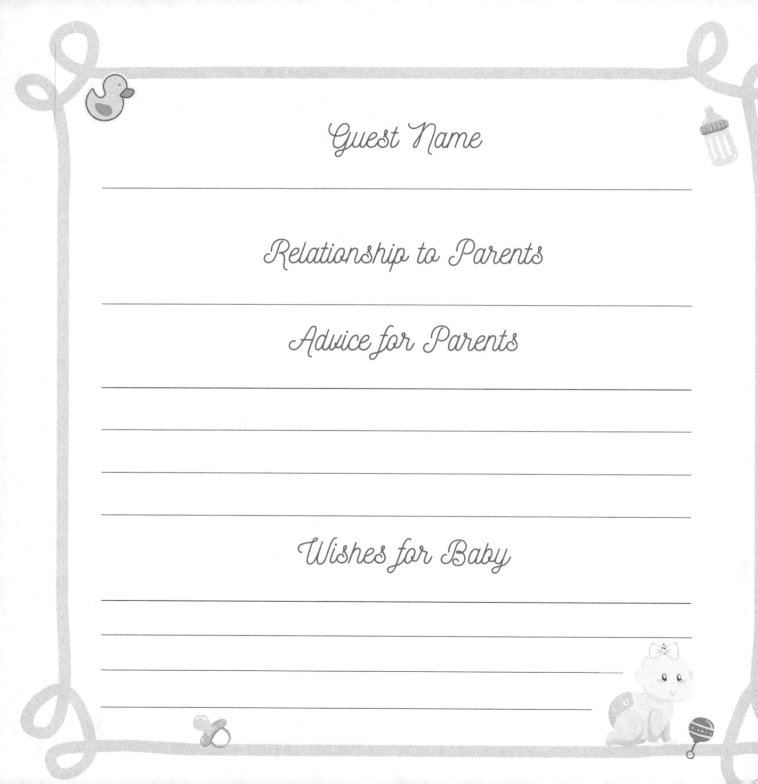

Guest Name

_____

Relationship to Parents

_____

Advice for Parents

_____

_____

_____

_____

Wishes for Baby

_____

_____

_____

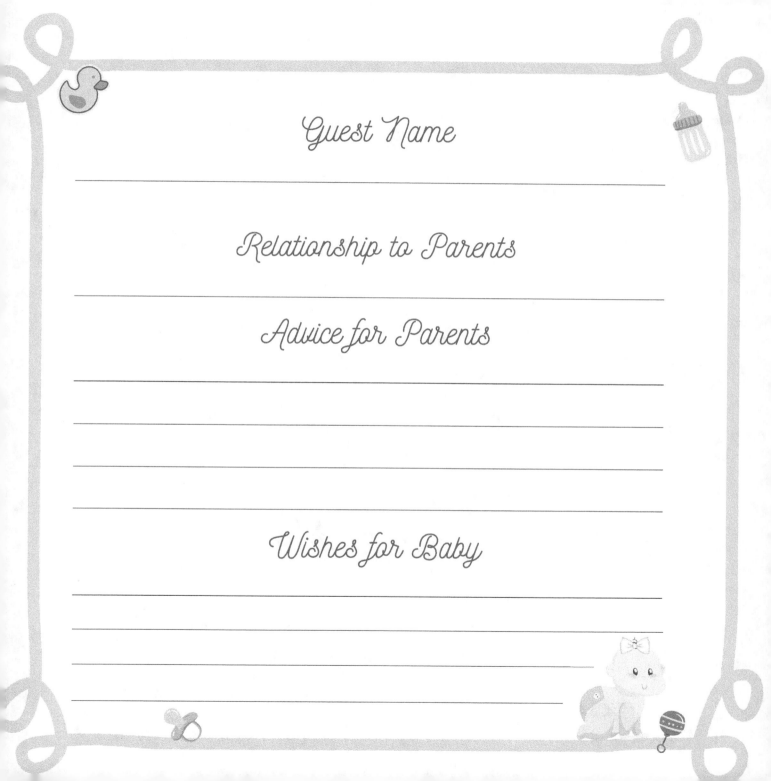

Guest Name

_____

Relationship to Parents

_____

Advice for Parents

_____

_____

_____

Wishes for Baby

_____

_____

_____

Guest Name

_____

Relationship to Parents

_____

Advice for Parents

_____

_____

_____

Wishes for Baby

_____

_____

_____

Guest Name

_____

Relationship to Parents

_____

Advice for Parents

_____

_____

_____

_____

Wishes for Baby

_____

_____

_____

Guest Name

_____

Relationship to Parents

_____

Advice for Parents

_____

_____

_____

Wishes for Baby

_____

_____

_____

Guest Name

_____

Relationship to Parents

_____

Advice for Parents

_____

_____

_____

Wishes for Baby

_____

_____

_____

Guest Name

_____

Relationship to Parents

_____

Advice for Parents

_____

_____

_____

Wishes for Baby

_____

_____

_____

Guest Name

_____

Relationship to Parents

_____

Advice for Parents

_____

_____

_____

Wishes for Baby

_____

_____

_____

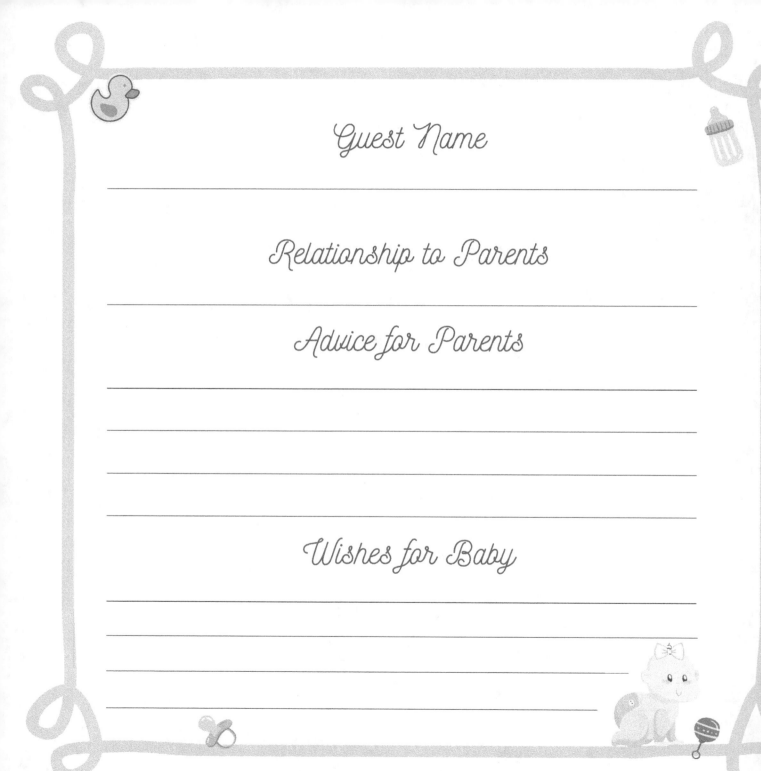

Guest Name

_____

Relationship to Parents

_____

Advice for Parents

_____

_____

_____

Wishes for Baby

_____

_____

_____

Guest Name

_____

Relationship to Parents

_____

Advice for Parents

_____

_____

_____

_____

Wishes for Baby

_____

_____

_____

_____

Guest Name

_____

Relationship to Parents

_____

Advice for Parents

_____

_____

_____

Wishes for Baby

_____

_____

_____

_____

Guest Name

_____

Relationship to Parents

_____

Advice for Parents

_____

_____

_____

_____

Wishes for Baby

_____

_____

_____

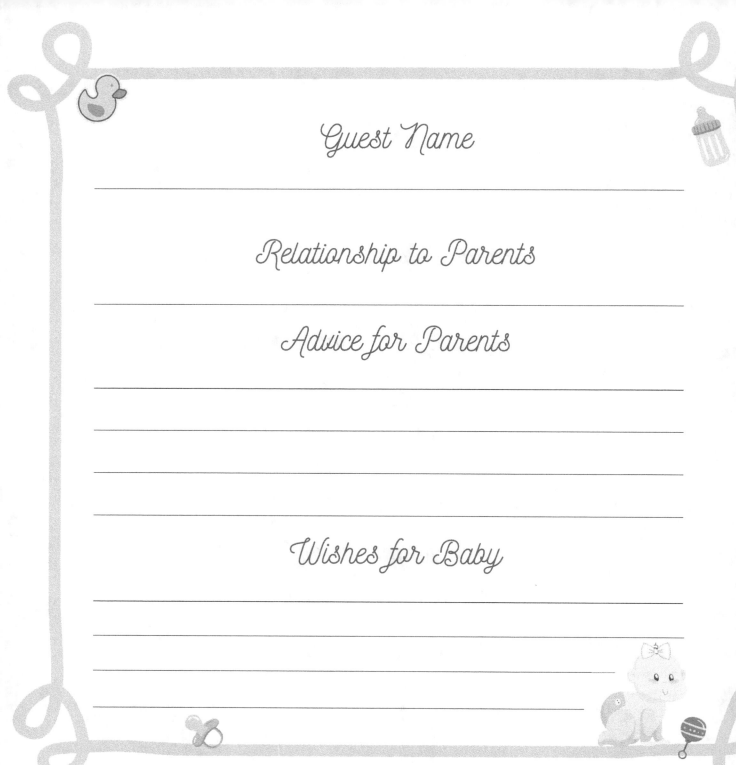

Guest Name

_____

Relationship to Parents

_____

Advice for Parents

_____

_____

_____

Wishes for Baby

_____

_____

_____

_____

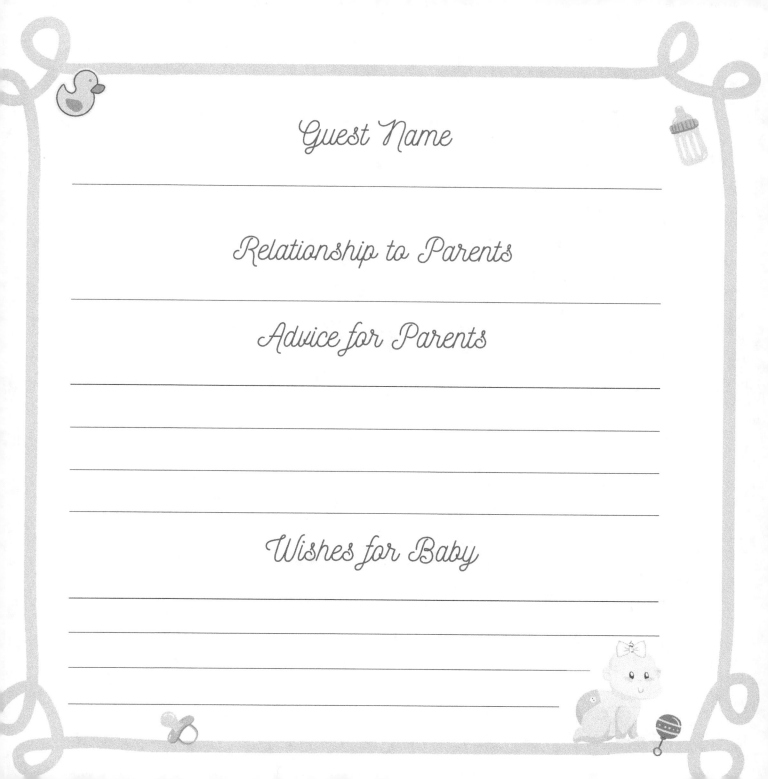

Guest Name

_____

Relationship to Parents

_____

Advice for Parents

_____

_____

_____

Wishes for Baby

_____

_____

_____

Guest Name

_____

Relationship to Parents

_____

Advice for Parents

_____

_____

_____

Wishes for Baby

_____

_____

_____

_____

Guest Name

_____

Relationship to Parents

_____

Advice for Parents

_____

_____

_____

_____

Wishes for Baby

_____

_____

_____

Guest Name

_____

Relationship to Parents

_____

Advice for Parents

_____

_____

_____

Wishes for Baby

_____

_____

_____

_____

Guest Name

_____

Relationship to Parents

_____

Advice for Parents

_____

_____

_____

_____

Wishes for Baby

_____

_____

_____

Guest Name

Relationship to Parents

Advice for Parents

Wishes for Baby

Guest Name

_____

Relationship to Parents

_____

Advice for Parents

_____

_____

_____

_____

Wishes for Baby

_____

_____

_____

_____

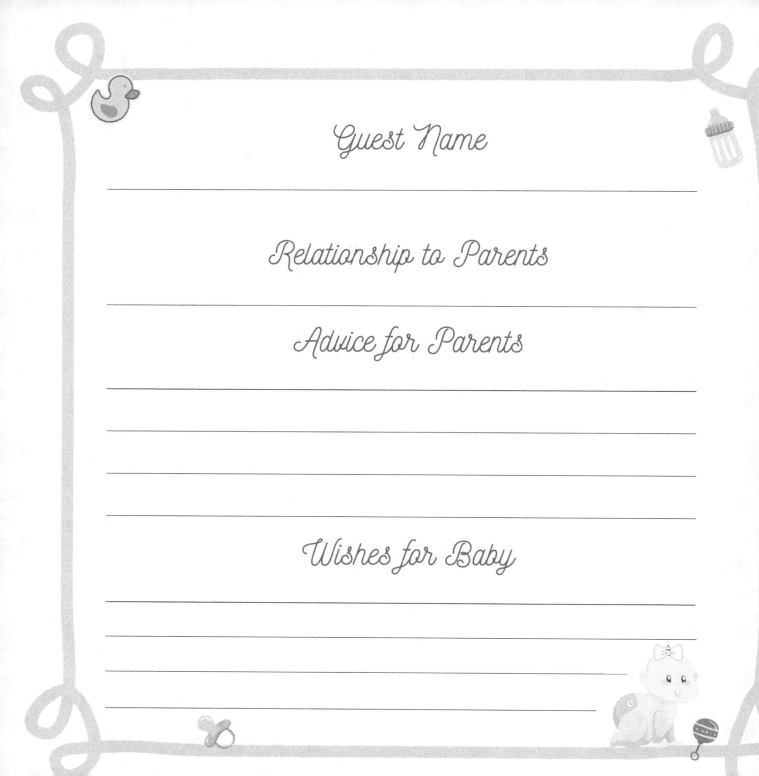

Guest Name

_____

Relationship to Parents

_____

Advice for Parents

_____

_____

_____

Wishes for Baby

_____

_____

_____

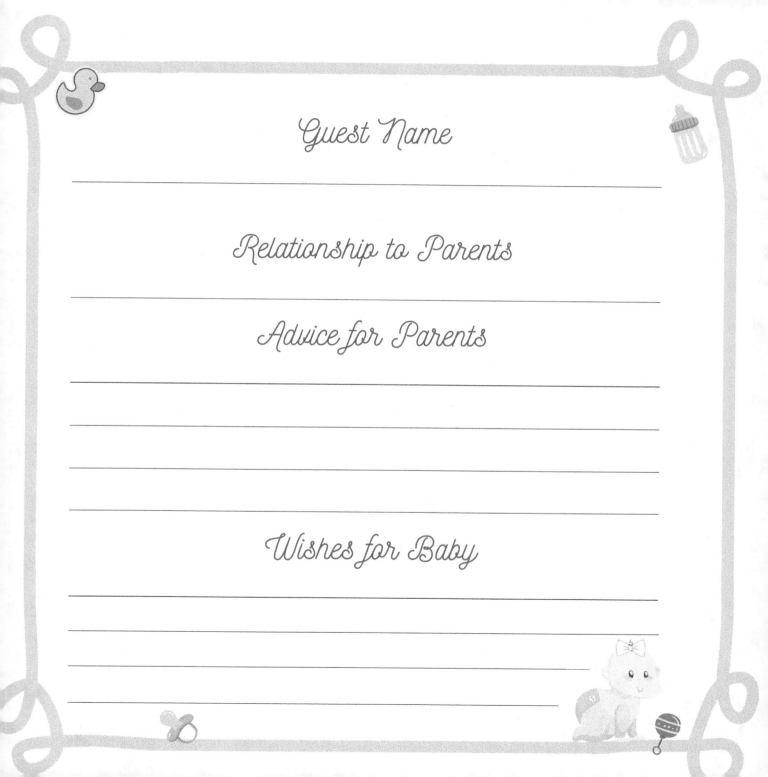

Guest Name

_____

Relationship to Parents

_____

Advice for Parents

_____

_____

_____

_____

Wishes for Baby

_____

_____

_____

_____

Guest Name

_____

Relationship to Parents

_____

Advice for Parents

_____

_____

_____

Wishes for Baby

_____

_____

_____

Guest Name

_____

Relationship to Parents

_____

Advice for Parents

_____

_____

_____

_____

Wishes for Baby

_____

_____

_____

_____

Guest Name

_____

Relationship to Parents

_____

Advice for Parents

_____

_____

_____

_____

Wishes for Baby

_____

_____

_____

_____

Guest Name

_____

Relationship to Parents

_____

Advice for Parents

_____

_____

_____

_____

Wishes for Baby

_____

_____

_____

Guest Name

_____

Relationship to Parents

_____

Advice for Parents

_____

_____

_____

Wishes for Baby

_____

_____

_____

Guest Name

_____

Relationship to Parents

_____

Advice for Parents

_____

_____

_____

_____

Wishes for Baby

_____

_____

_____

Guest Name

_____

Relationship to Parents

_____

Advice for Parents

_____

_____

_____

Wishes for Baby

_____

_____

_____

Guest Name

_____

Relationship to Parents

_____

Advice for Parents

_____

_____

_____

_____

Wishes for Baby

_____

_____

_____

_____

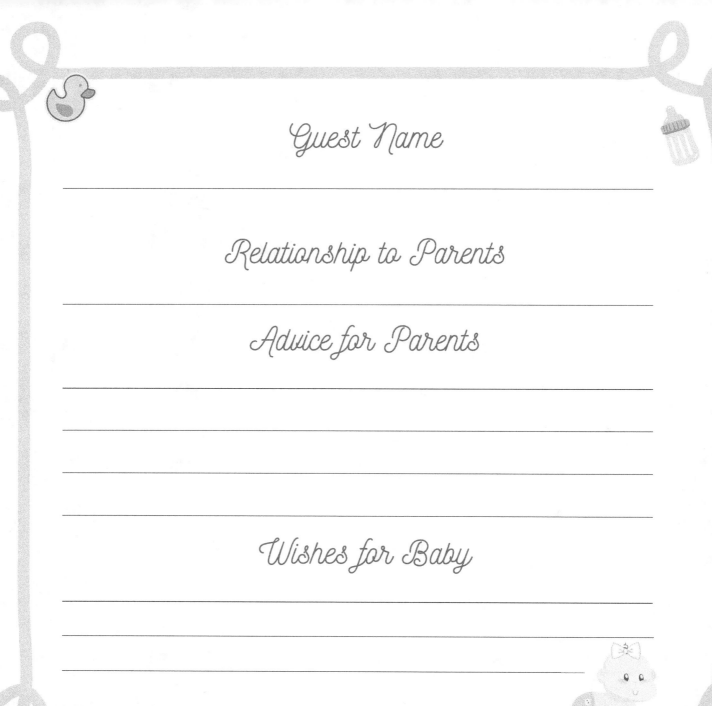

Guest Name

_____

Relationship to Parents

_____

Advice for Parents

_____

_____

_____

_____

Wishes for Baby

_____

_____

_____

Guest Name

_____

Relationship to Parents

_____

Advice for Parents

_____

_____

_____

_____

Wishes for Baby

_____

_____

_____

Guest Name

_____

Relationship to Parents

_____

Advice for Parents

_____

_____

_____

Wishes for Baby

_____

_____

_____

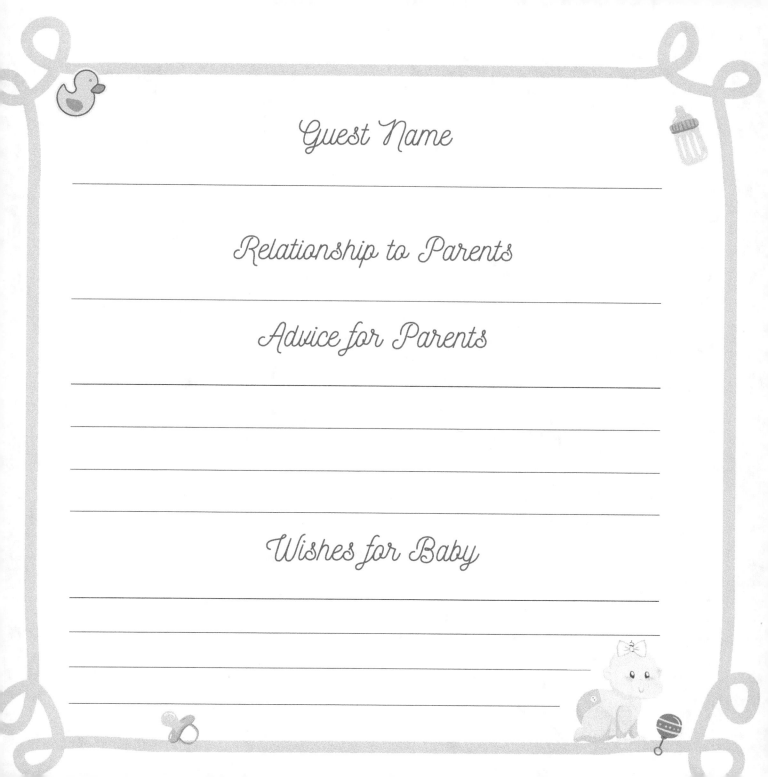

Guest Name

_____

Relationship to Parents

_____

Advice for Parents

_____

_____

_____

_____

Wishes for Baby

_____

_____

_____

_____

Guest Name

_____

Relationship to Parents

_____

Advice for Parents

_____

_____

_____

Wishes for Baby

_____

_____

_____

Guest Name

_____

Relationship to Parents

_____

Advice for Parents

_____

_____

_____

Wishes for Baby

_____

_____

_____

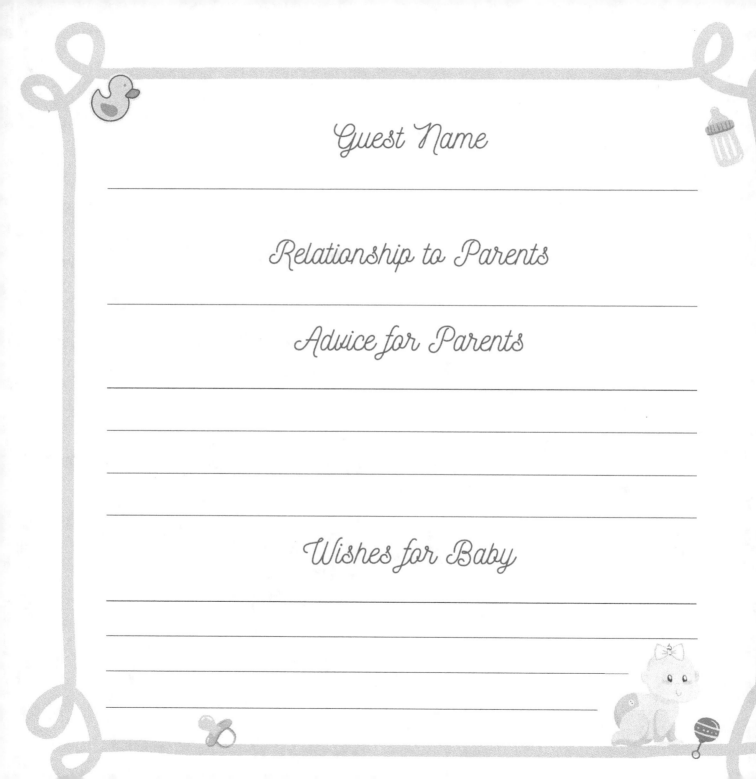

Guest Name

_____

Relationship to Parents

_____

Advice for Parents

_____

_____

_____

Wishes for Baby

_____

_____

_____

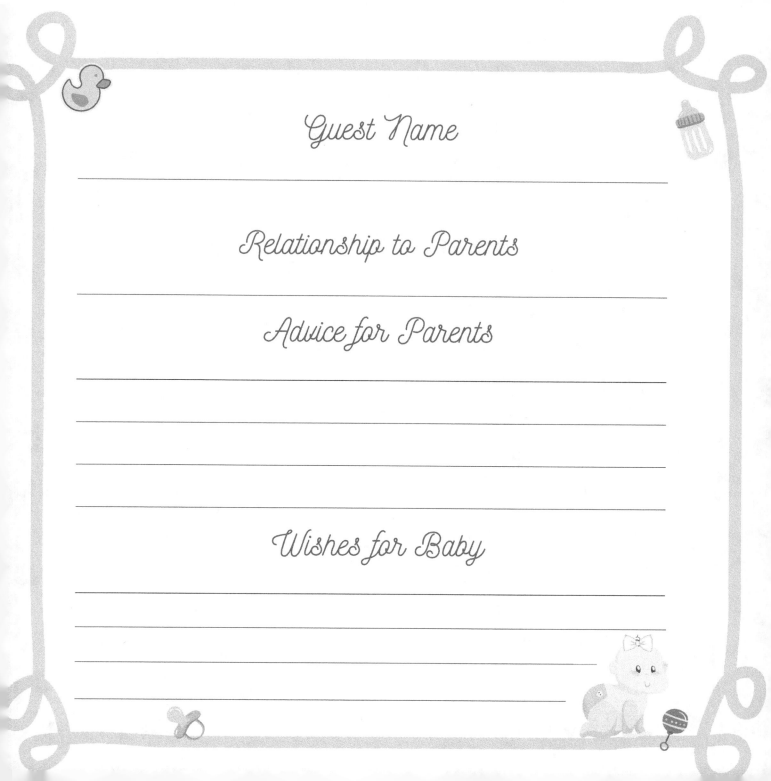

Guest Name

_____

Relationship to Parents

_____

Advice for Parents

_____

_____

_____

_____

Wishes for Baby

_____

_____

_____

_____

Guest Name

_____

Relationship to Parents

_____

Advice for Parents

_____

_____

_____

Wishes for Baby

_____

_____

_____

Guest Name

_____

Relationship to Parents

_____

Advice for Parents

_____

_____

_____

_____

Wishes for Baby

_____

_____

_____

_____

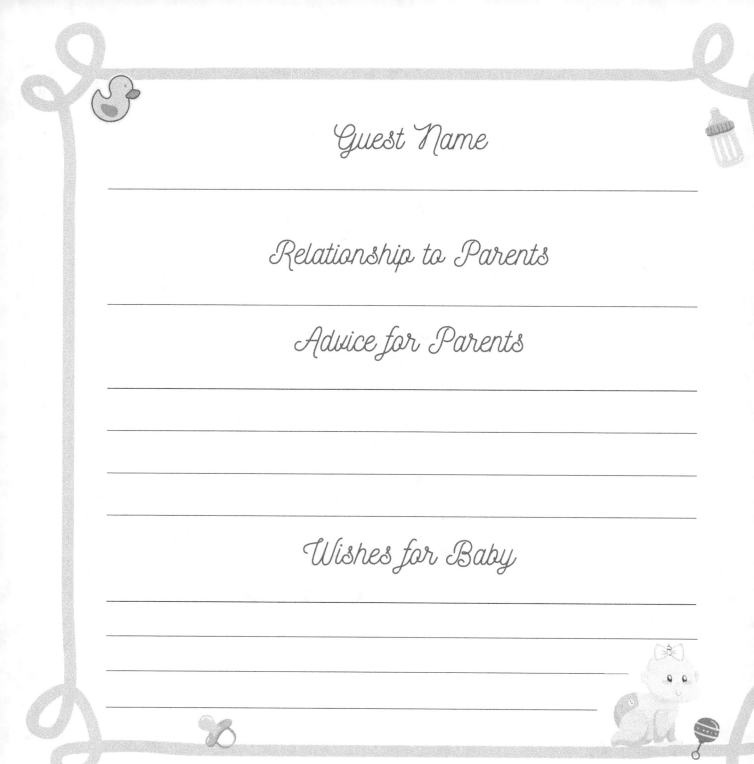

Guest Name

_____

Relationship to Parents

_____

Advice for Parents

_____

_____

_____

Wishes for Baby

_____

_____

_____

Guest Name

_____

Relationship to Parents

_____

Advice for Parents

_____

_____

_____

_____

Wishes for Baby

_____

_____

_____

_____

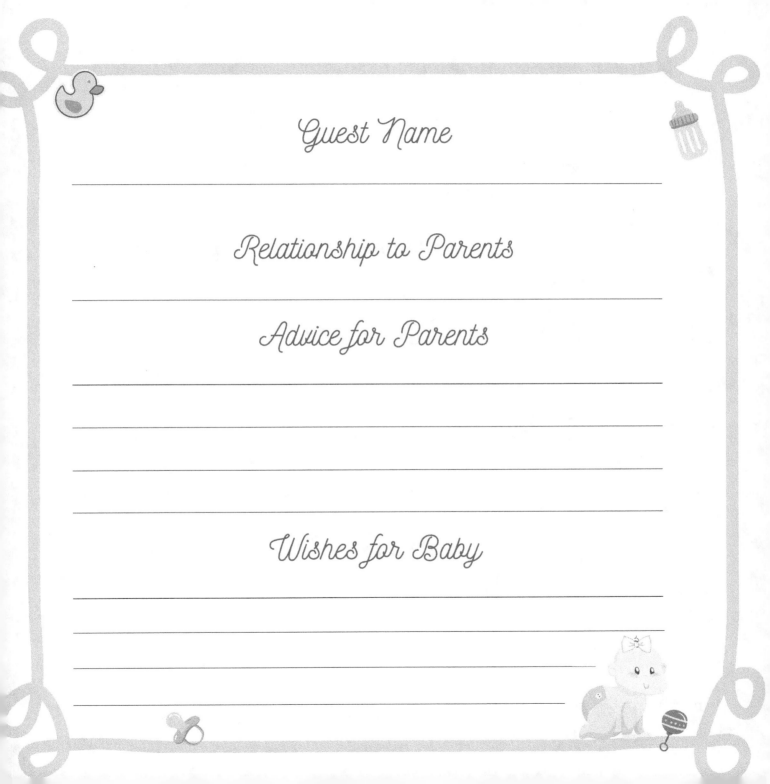

Guest Name

_____

Relationship to Parents

_____

Advice for Parents

_____

_____

_____

Wishes for Baby

_____

_____

_____

Guest Name

_____

Relationship to Parents

_____

Advice for Parents

_____

_____

_____

Wishes for Baby

_____

_____

_____

Guest Name

_____

Relationship to Parents

_____

Advice for Parents

_____

_____

_____

Wishes for Baby

_____

_____

_____

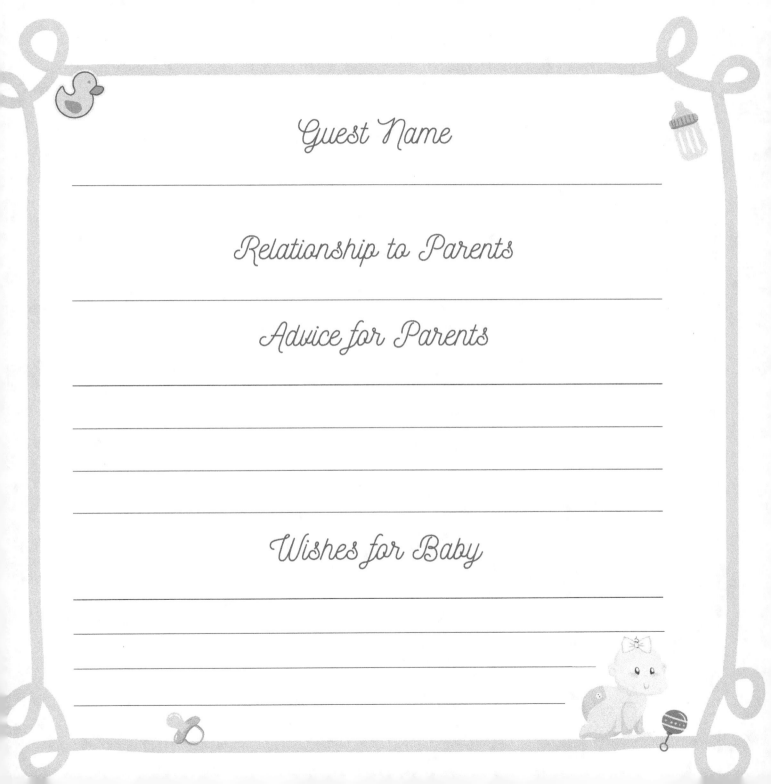

Guest Name

_____

Relationship to Parents

_____

Advice for Parents

_____

_____

_____

Wishes for Baby

_____

_____

_____

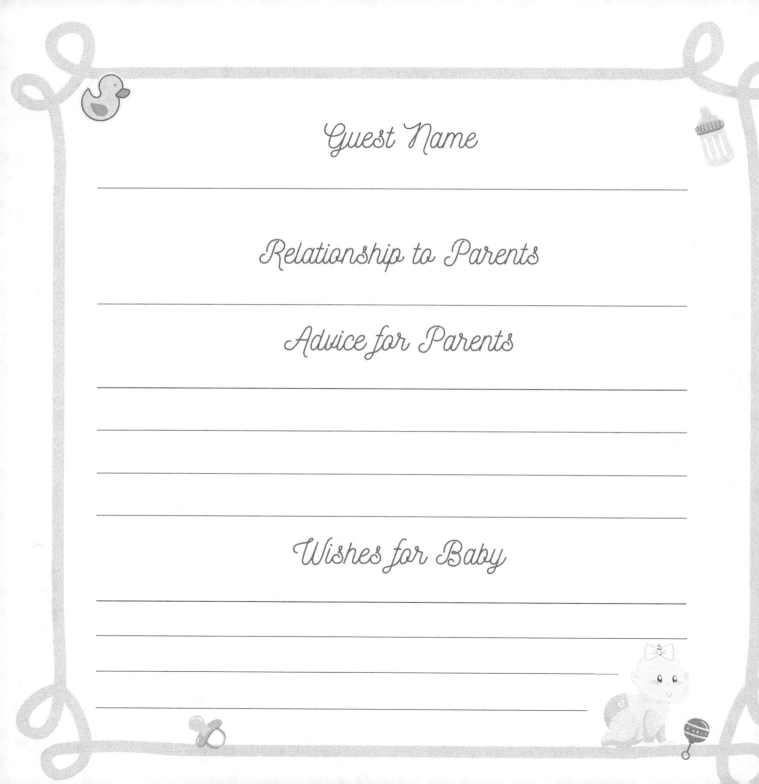

Guest Name

_____

Relationship to Parents

_____

Advice for Parents

_____

_____

_____

_____

Wishes for Baby

_____

_____

_____

_____

Guest Name

_____

Relationship to Parents

_____

Advice for Parents

_____

_____

_____

_____

Wishes for Baby

_____

_____

_____

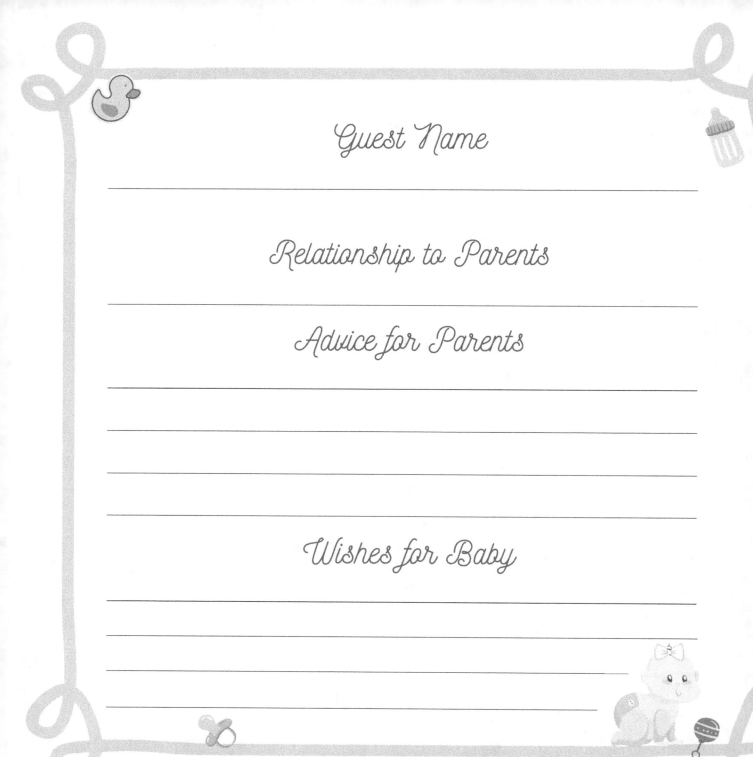

Guest Name

_____

Relationship to Parents

_____

Advice for Parents

_____

_____

_____

Wishes for Baby

_____

_____

_____

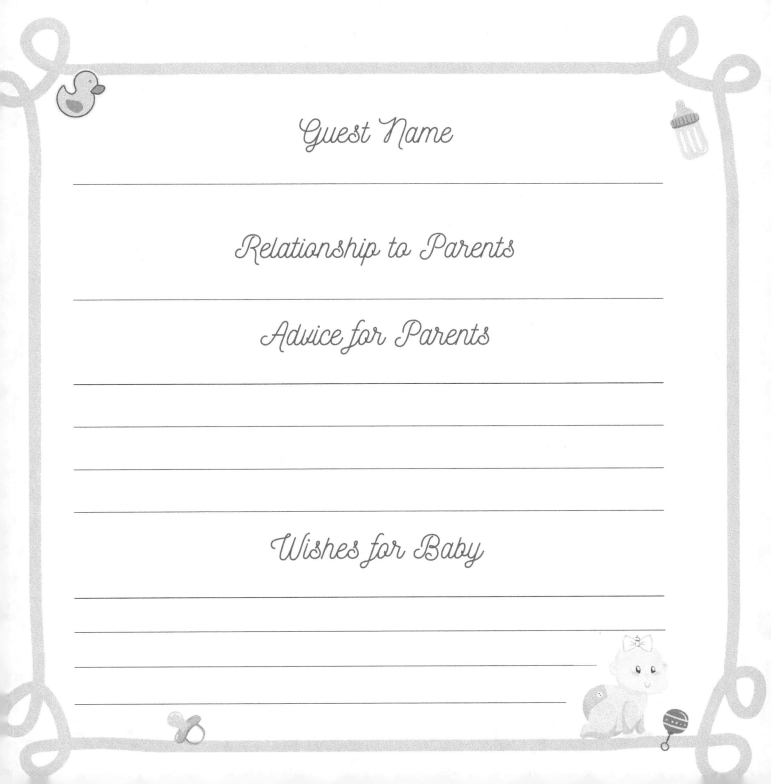

Guest Name

_____

Relationship to Parents

_____

Advice for Parents

_____

_____

_____

_____

Wishes for Baby

_____

_____

_____

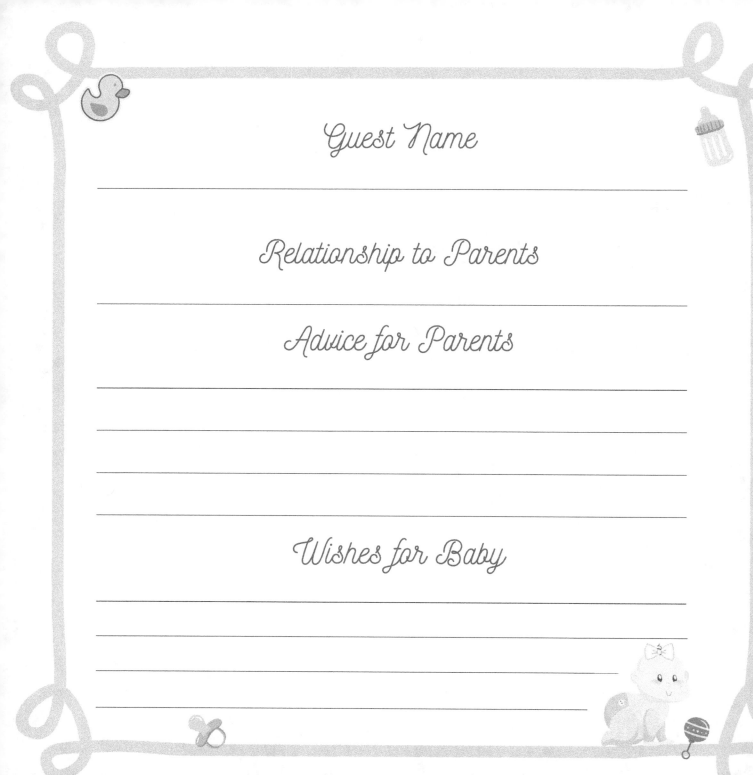

Guest Name

_____

Relationship to Parents

_____

Advice for Parents

_____

_____

_____

Wishes for Baby

_____

_____

_____

_____

Guest Name

_____

Relationship to Parents

_____

Advice for Parents

_____

_____

_____

_____

Wishes for Baby

_____

_____

_____

Guest Name

_____

Relationship to Parents

_____

Advice for Parents

_____

_____

_____

Wishes for Baby

_____

_____

_____

Guest Name

_____

Relationship to Parents

_____

Advice for Parents

_____

_____

_____

_____

Wishes for Baby

_____

_____

_____

Guest Name

_____

Relationship to Parents

_____

Advice for Parents

_____

_____

_____

Wishes for Baby

_____

_____

_____

Guest Name

_____

Relationship to Parents

_____

Advice for Parents

_____

_____

_____

_____

Wishes for Baby

_____

_____

_____

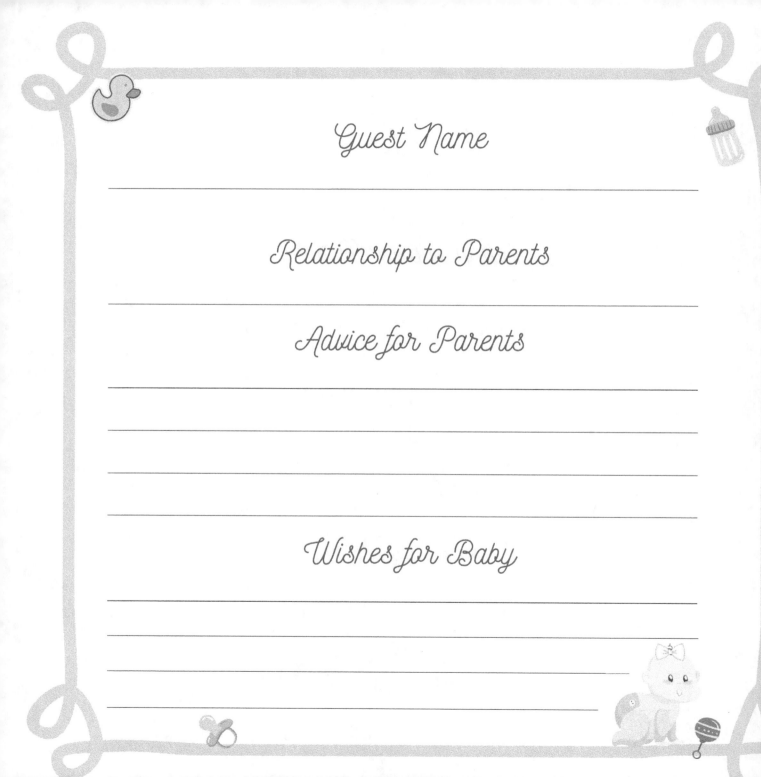

Guest Name

_____

Relationship to Parents

_____

Advice for Parents

_____

_____

_____

Wishes for Baby

_____

_____

_____

Guest Name

_____

Relationship to Parents

_____

Advice for Parents

_____

_____

_____

_____

Wishes for Baby

_____

_____

_____

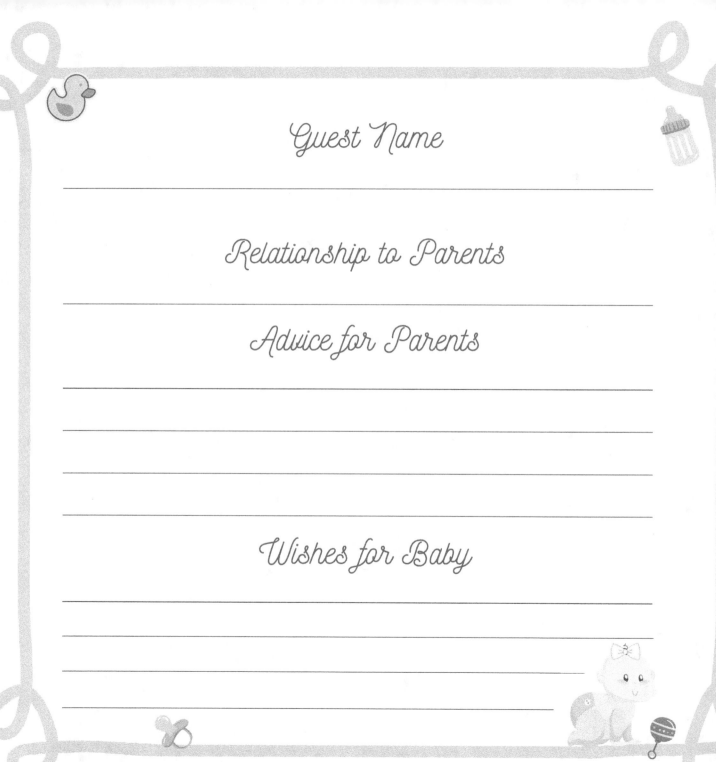

Guest Name

_____

Relationship to Parents

_____

Advice for Parents

_____

_____

_____

Wishes for Baby

_____

_____

_____

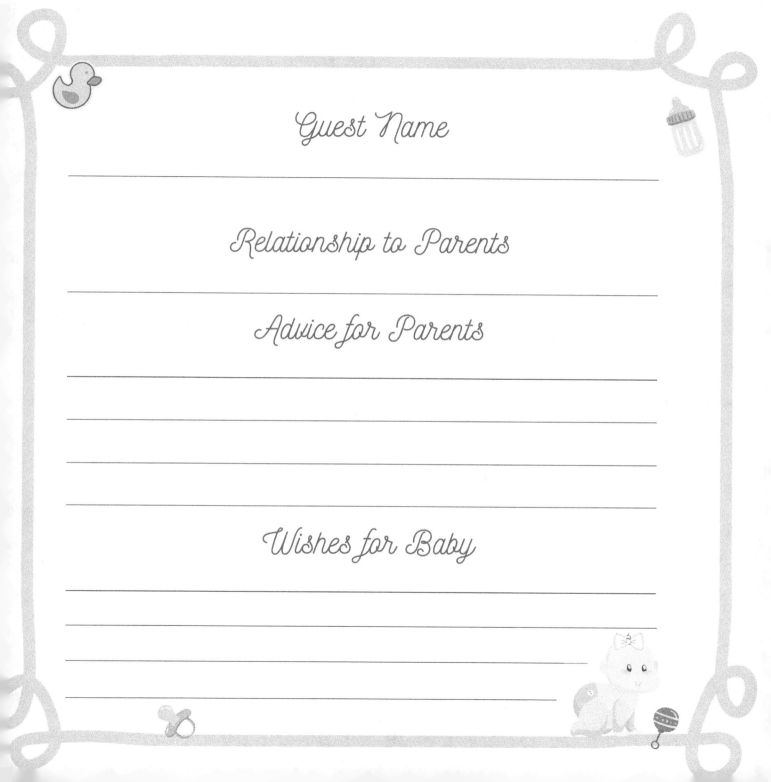

Guest Name

_____

Relationship to Parents

_____

Advice for Parents

_____

_____

_____

_____

Wishes for Baby

_____

_____

_____

Guest Name

_____

Relationship to Parents

_____

Advice for Parents

_____

_____

_____

Wishes for Baby

_____

_____

_____

Guest Name

_____

Relationship to Parents

_____

Advice for Parents

_____

_____

_____

_____

Wishes for Baby

_____

_____

_____

_____

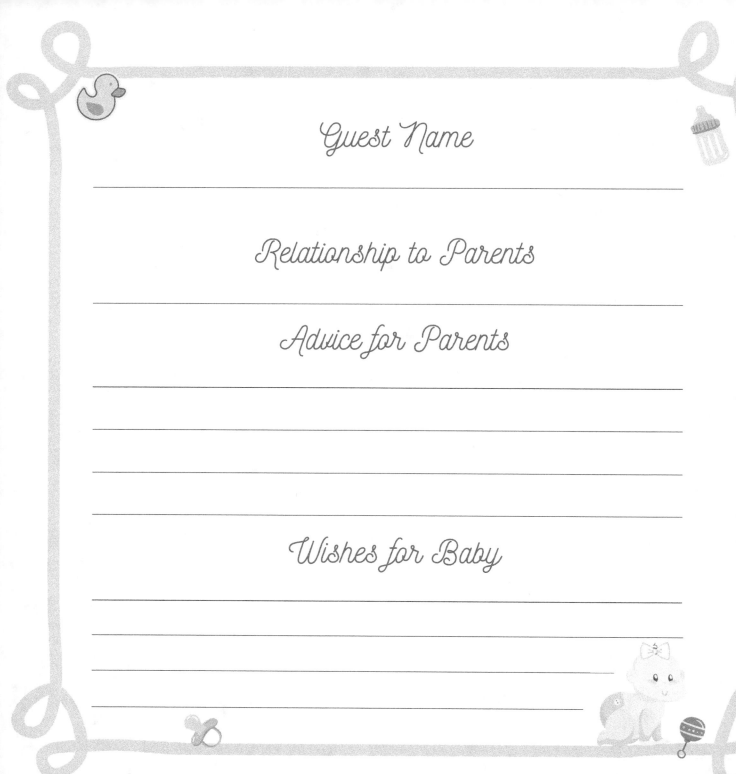

Guest Name

_____

Relationship to Parents

_____

Advice for Parents

_____

_____

_____

Wishes for Baby

_____

_____

_____

Guest Name

_____

Relationship to Parents

_____

Advice for Parents

_____

_____

_____

_____

Wishes for Baby

_____

_____

_____

_____

Guest Name

_____

Relationship to Parents

_____

Advice for Parents

_____

_____

_____

_____

Wishes for Baby

_____

_____

_____

_____

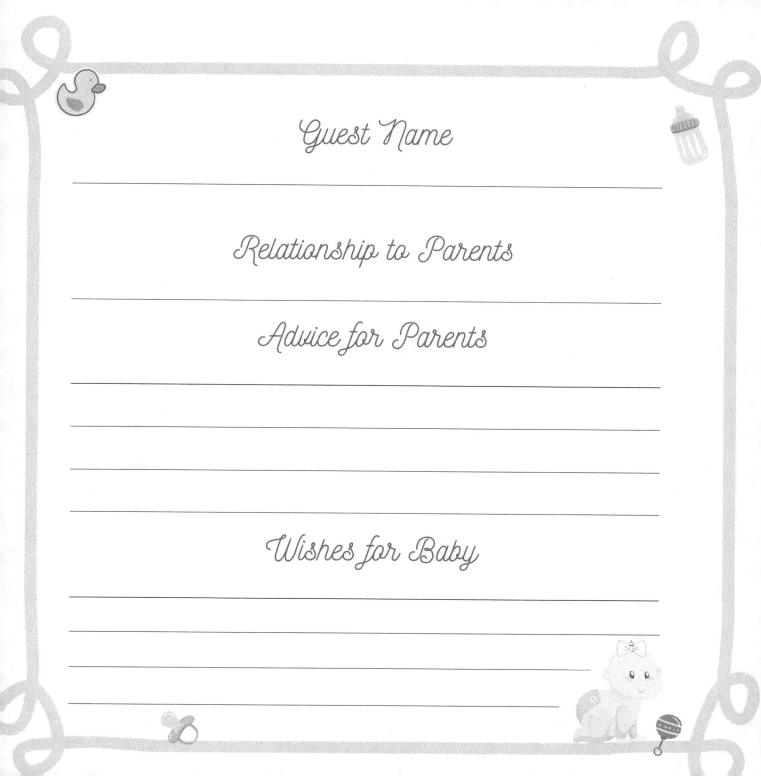

Guest Name

_____

Relationship to Parents

_____

Advice for Parents

_____

_____

_____

Wishes for Baby

_____

_____

_____

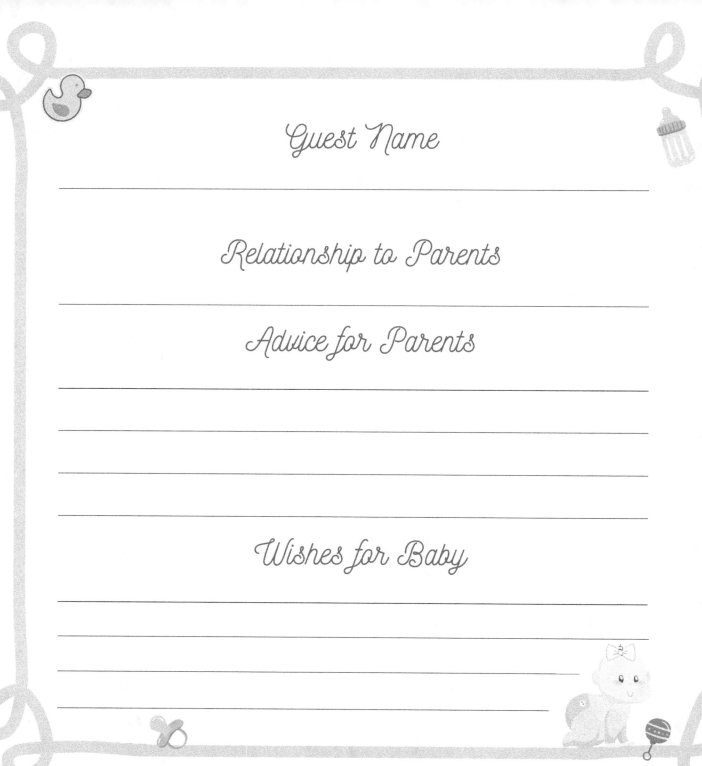

Guest Name

_____

Relationship to Parents

_____

Advice for Parents

_____

_____

_____

Wishes for Baby

_____

_____

_____

Guest Name

_____

Relationship to Parents

_____

Advice for Parents

_____

_____

_____

_____

Wishes for Baby

_____

_____

_____

_____

Guest Name

_____

Relationship to Parents

_____

Advice for Parents

_____

_____

_____

Wishes for Baby

_____

_____

_____

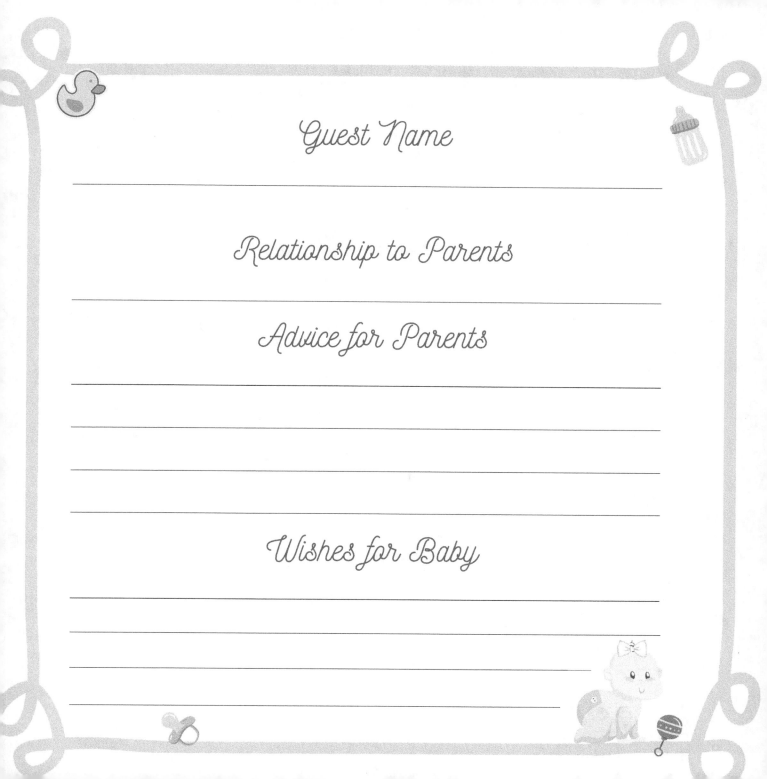

Guest Name

_____

Relationship to Parents

_____

Advice for Parents

_____

_____

_____

_____

Wishes for Baby

_____

_____

_____

Guest Name

_____

Relationship to Parents

_____

Advice for Parents

_____

_____

_____

_____

Wishes for Baby

_____

_____

_____

_____

Guest Name

_____

Relationship to Parents

_____

Advice for Parents

_____

_____

_____

_____

Wishes for Baby

_____

_____

_____

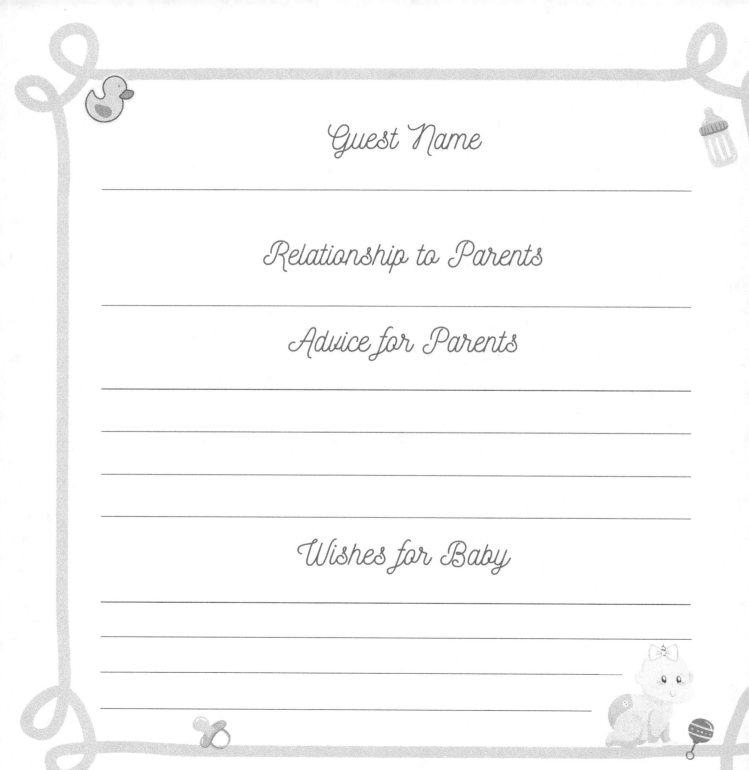

Guest Name

_____

Relationship to Parents

_____

Advice for Parents

_____

_____

_____

Wishes for Baby

_____

_____

_____

Guest Name

_____

Relationship to Parents

_____

Advice for Parents

_____

_____

_____

_____

Wishes for Baby

_____

_____

_____

Guest Name

_____

Relationship to Parents

_____

Advice for Parents

_____

_____

_____

Wishes for Baby

_____

_____

_____

Guest Name

_____

Relationship to Parents

_____

Advice for Parents

_____

_____

_____

_____

Wishes for Baby

_____

_____

_____

_____

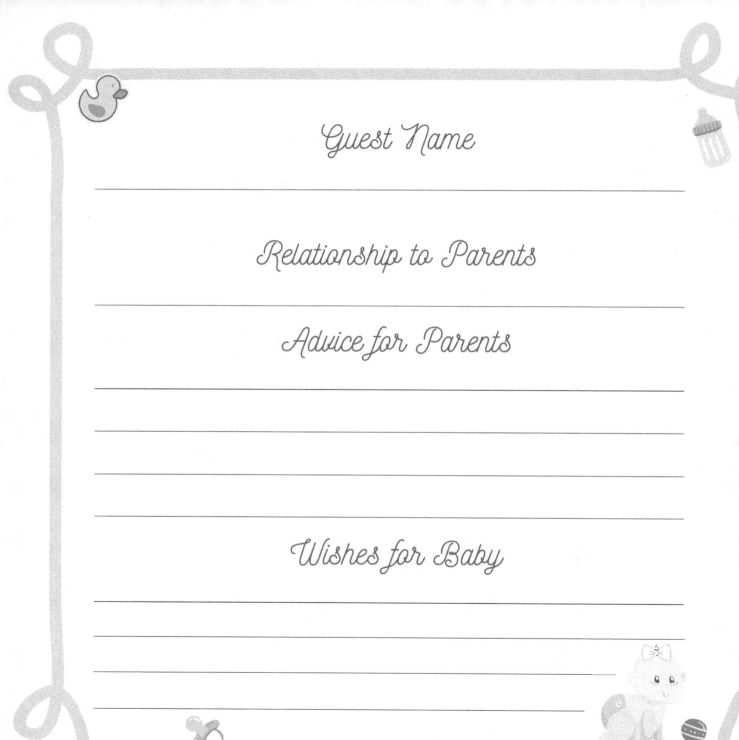

Guest Name

_____

Relationship to Parents

_____

Advice for Parents

_____

_____

_____

Wishes for Baby

_____

_____

_____

_____

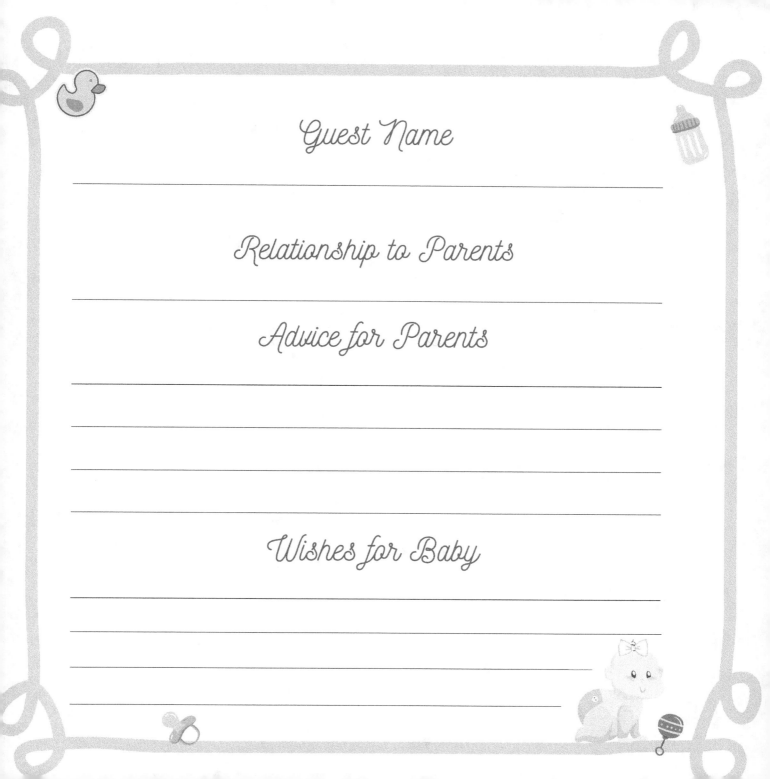

Guest Name

_____

Relationship to Parents

_____

Advice for Parents

_____

_____

_____

_____

Wishes for Baby

_____

_____

_____

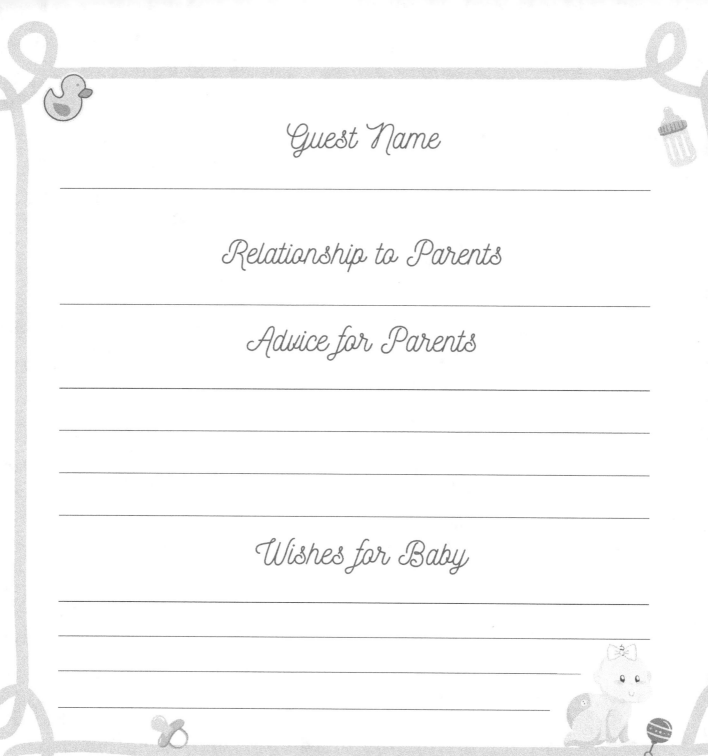

Guest Name

_____

Relationship to Parents

_____

Advice for Parents

_____

_____

_____

Wishes for Baby

_____

_____

_____

Guest Name

_____

Relationship to Parents

_____

Advice for Parents

_____

_____

_____

Wishes for Baby

_____

_____

_____

Guest Name

_____

Relationship to Parents

_____

Advice for Parents

_____

_____

_____

Wishes for Baby

_____

_____

_____

Guest Name

_____

Relationship to Parents

_____

Advice for Parents

_____

_____

_____

_____

Wishes for Baby

_____

_____

_____

_____

Guest Name

Relationship to Parents

Advice for Parents

Wishes for Baby

Guest Name

_____

Relationship to Parents

_____

Advice for Parents

_____

_____

_____

Wishes for Baby

_____

_____

_____

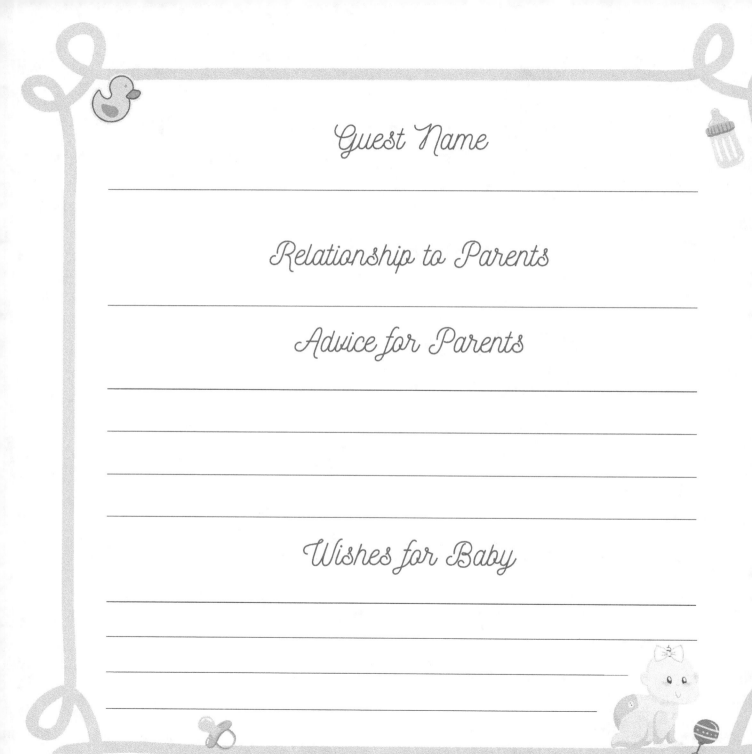

Guest Name

_____

Relationship to Parents

_____

Advice for Parents

_____

_____

_____

Wishes for Baby

_____

_____

_____

Guest Name

_____

Relationship to Parents

_____

Advice for Parents

_____

_____

_____

Wishes for Baby

_____

_____

_____

Guest Name

_____

Relationship to Parents

_____

Advice for Parents

_____

_____

_____

Wishes for Baby

_____

_____

_____

_____

Guest Name

_____

Relationship to Parents

_____

Advice for Parents

_____

_____

_____

_____

Wishes for Baby

_____

_____

_____

_____

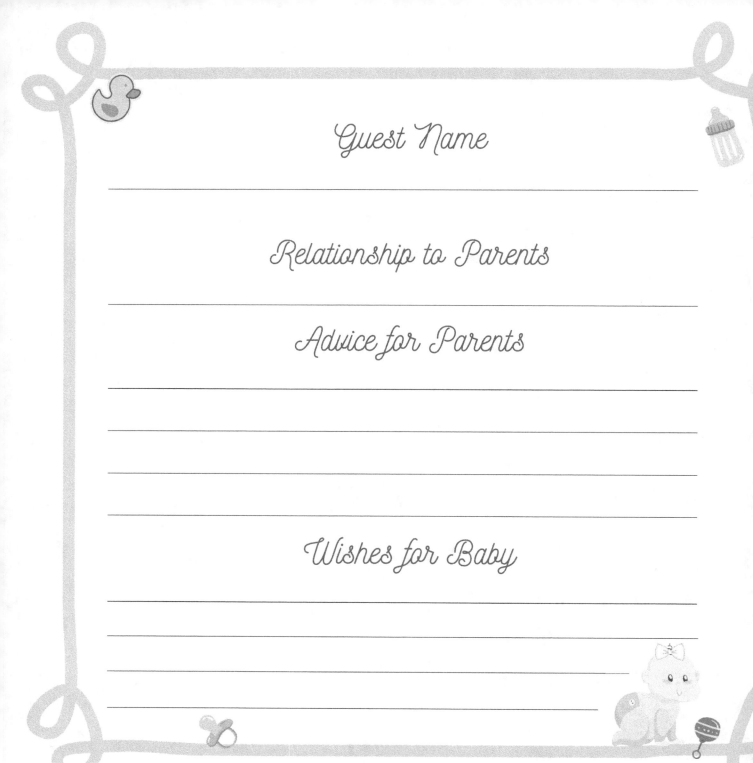

Guest Name

_____

Relationship to Parents

_____

Advice for Parents

_____

_____

_____

Wishes for Baby

_____

_____

_____

Guest Name

_____

Relationship to Parents

_____

Advice for Parents

_____

_____

_____

Wishes for Baby

_____

_____

_____

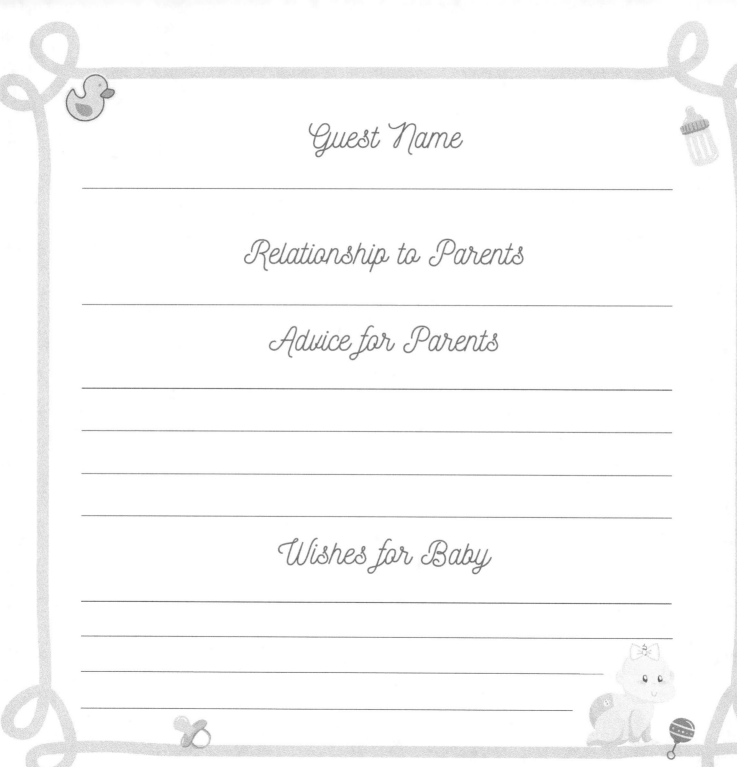

Guest Name

_____

Relationship to Parents

_____

Advice for Parents

_____

_____

_____

Wishes for Baby

_____

_____

_____

Guest Name

_____

Relationship to Parents

_____

Advice for Parents

_____

_____

_____

_____

Wishes for Baby

_____

_____

_____

Guest Name

_____

Relationship to Parents

_____

Advice for Parents

_____

_____

_____

Wishes for Baby

_____

_____

_____

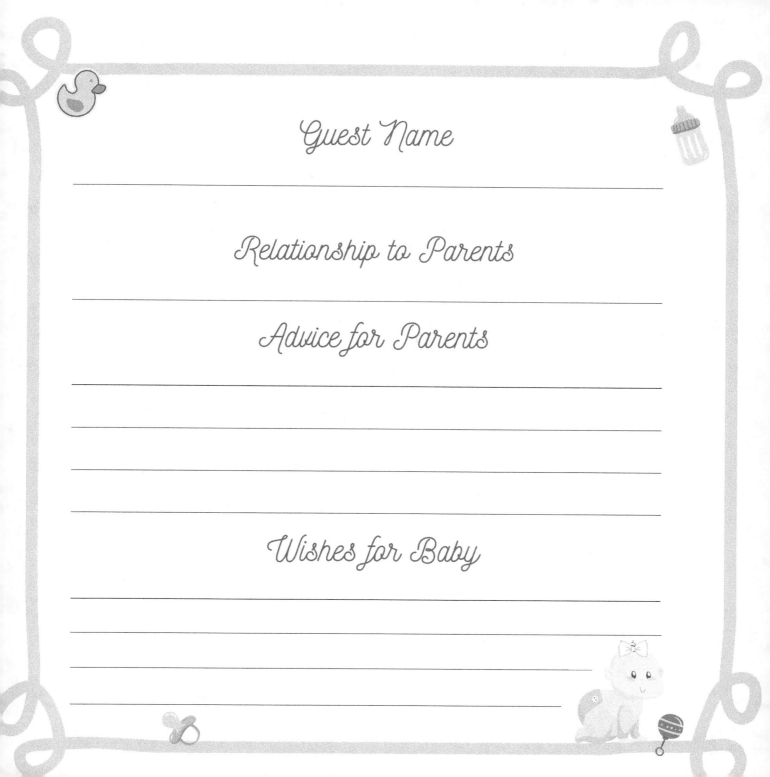

Guest Name

_____

Relationship to Parents

_____

Advice for Parents

_____

_____

_____

_____

Wishes for Baby

_____

_____

_____

Guest Name

_____

Relationship to Parents

_____

Advice for Parents

_____

_____

_____

_____

Wishes for Baby

_____

_____

_____

_____

Notes / Photos

Notes / Photos

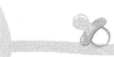

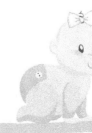

Notes / Photos

Notes / Photos

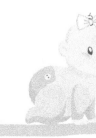

Notes / Photos

Notes / Photos

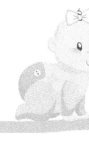

Notes / Photos

Notes / Photos

Gift Log

Name/Email/Phone

Gift

_____   _____

_____   _____

_____   _____

_____   _____

_____   _____

_____   _____

_____   _____

_____   _____

_____   _____

_____   _____

_____   _____

_____   _____

_____   _____

Gift Log

Name/Email/Phone	Gift
_____	_____
_____	_____
_____	_____
_____	_____
_____	_____
_____	_____
_____	_____
_____	_____
_____	_____
_____	_____
_____	_____
_____	_____
_____	_____
_____	_____

Gift Log

Name/Email/Phone	Gift
_____	_____
_____	_____
_____	_____
_____	_____
_____	_____
_____	_____
_____	_____
_____	_____
_____	_____
_____	_____
_____	_____
_____	_____
_____	_____
_____	_____

Gift Log

Name/Email/Phone	Gift
_____	_____
_____	_____
_____	_____
_____	_____
_____	_____
_____	_____
_____	_____
_____	_____
_____	_____
_____	_____
_____	_____
_____	_____
_____	_____

Gift Log

Name/Email/Phone

Gift

_____

_____

_____

_____

_____

_____

_____

_____

_____

_____

_____

_____

_____

Gift Log

Name/Email/Phone	Gift

Gift Log

Name/Email/Phone	Gift
_____	_____
_____	_____
_____	_____
_____	_____
_____	_____
_____	_____
_____	_____
_____	_____
_____	_____
_____	_____
_____	_____
_____	_____
_____	_____
_____	_____

Gift Log

Name/Email/Phone	Gift

Gift Log

Name/Email/Phone   Gift

_____   _____

_____   _____

_____   _____

_____   _____

_____   _____

_____   _____

_____   _____

_____   _____

_____   _____

_____   _____

_____   _____

_____   _____

_____   _____

_____   _____

Gift Log

Name/Email/Phone	Gift

Printed in the USA
CPSIA information can be obtained
at www.ICGtesting.com
LVHW080716161023
761141LV00037B/70